THE DOG THAT DIDN'T GIVE UP

PUBLISHED by Be Romantic Publishing Co. also known as B.R. Publishing
1725 Pinebrook Dr.
Knoxville, TN 37909
(423) 691-1990

ISBN#0-9625593-3-4

WRITTEN by Barry Rosen
ILLUSTRATIONS by Greg Bell *(Greg is for hire contact B.R. Publishing Co.)*

SECOND EDITION

Some of the money from this book will go to feed hungrey kids in the United States. If you would like to help feed kids please send your check to : **Kid Care, P.O. Box 92025, Houston Tx 77206.** They won The President Award, The Quaker Award and were The Person of the week on ABC News for more information call (713) 695-5437

This is based on a true story. The people are made into dogs to make it more fun to read. The story is about a dog named Bear. Bear lived on a planet where dogs and cats could talk just like people do on earth.

When Bear was a puppy his mom was trying to teach him how to count to ten. After a few weeks of hard work, Bear finally did it. He could count to ten without any help from his mom. He was so happy he would walk up to other dogs and cats and then start counting for them. Bear felt that he was the smartest puppy on the planet. He liked other dogs and cats to think that he was smart, too.

Till one day he walked up to other puppies his age, and found out that they could also count to ten. Bear learned that he was not the smartest puppy on the planet. He was just as smart as all the rest of the puppies his age.

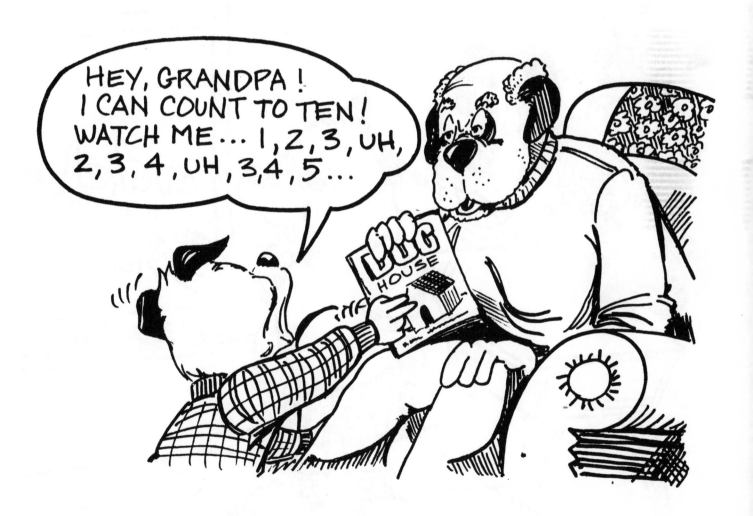

The next year Bear started to go to school. The first thing they learned was how to say their ABC's. That's when the other dogs started making fun of Bear for putting the round part of some letters backwards. The teacher asked Bear to go up to the blackboard, and write his ABC's. Bear started to write a d c b, when some of the dogs started to howl. Howling to a dog is the same as laughing is to a human. Bear kept on writing e f g h i j k l n m. Some more dogs howled as he wrote o q p r s t v u w x y z. Bear was putting letters down backwards-like b he would put d, n he would put m, p he was putting q and u he put v. By the time Bear was done, all the dogs started to howl at him. One dog even called Bear stupid for not knowing his ABC's.

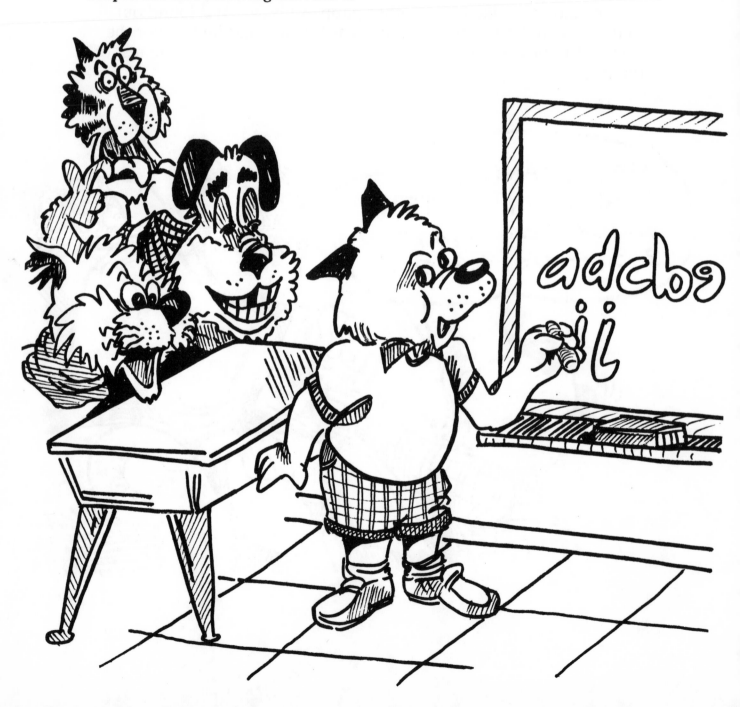

Bear ran out of the classroom with his head down and his tail between his legs yelling "I'M NOT STUPID I'M NOT DUMB ONE DAY I WILL SHOW YOU I WILL BE FAMOUS AND WE WILL SEE WHO IS HOWLING THEN"!

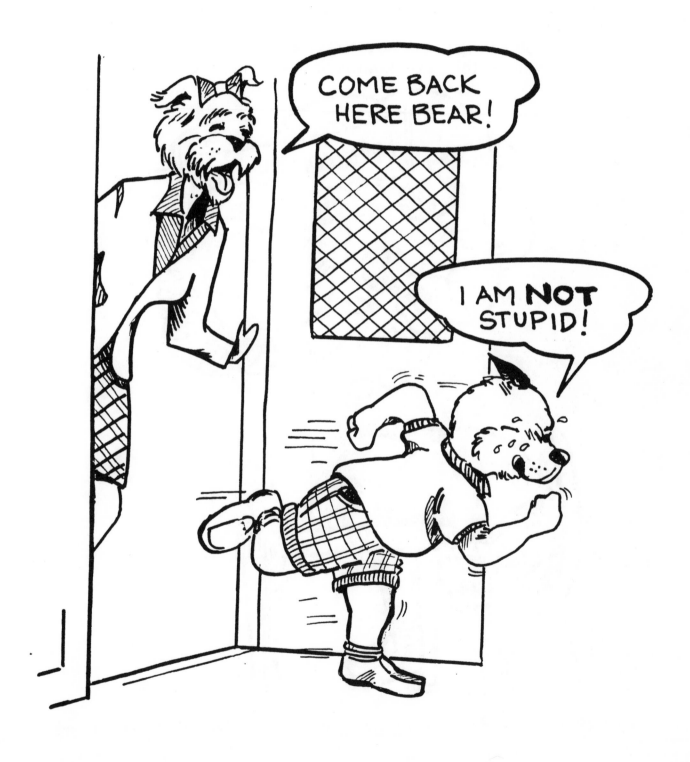

Bear now had a dream, a goal to be famous. He didn't know how he was going to be famous, but he was going to do it and show everyone he was a special dog.

Even though the other dogs and cats were making fun of him, Bear was very smart. His IQ was above normal, but at that time Bear didn't know he had a learning problem known as DYSLEXIA (dys-lex-ia). Dyslexia is when you will reverse letters or numbers thinking you are doing it right. It also affects the way you read and do math because you see things backwards or words that are not there.

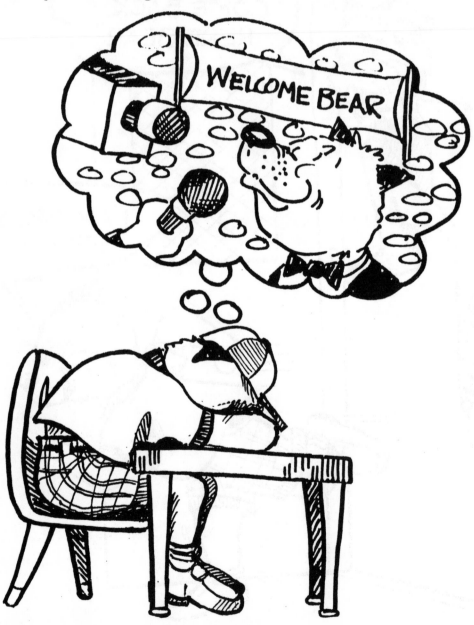

DYSLEXIA: Is when a person can't read do to an unknown reason

That same year Bear had to learn to say the Pledge of Allegiance(al-le-giance) to the flag. When saying the Pledge of Allegiance, they had to put their right paw on their chest. Bear would get mixed up, and he would forget which paw was his right, and which one was his left. Even though they did it every day he couldn't remember it. He would have to wait to see which paw the other dogs would put up before he would put his paw up, so that the other dogs wouldn't howl at him. Bear didn't like it when the other dogs were howling at him. It made him feel like he was not as smart as the rest of the dogs.

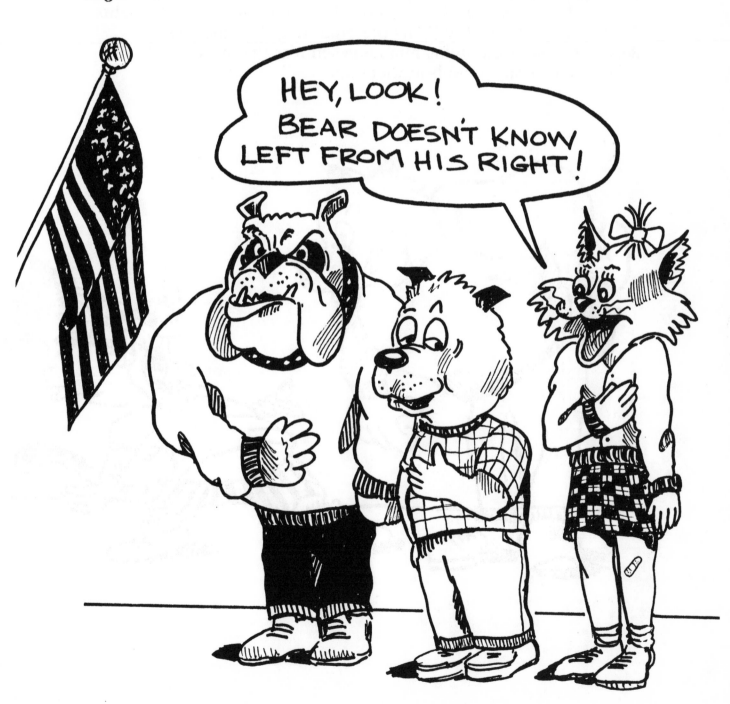

The next year the dogs started to learn how to read. Bear had very few problems with making the sound of each letter. Where he did have the problem was putting the sounds together. When he had two or more sounds together he would get the sounds mixed up. He just didn't understand how sounds went together.

Bear was getting behind in reading. The dogs started to make fun of him. Bear started to get mad. So, in order to stop the other dogs from making fun of him, and calling him names, Bear would have dog fights with the other dogs, and cats. Bear was much bigger than the other dogs and cats in his class. He would always win the fights. After Bear got into a few fights the other dogs became afraid of Bear. They stopped calling him names in fear that if they did call him a name, Bear would beat them up.

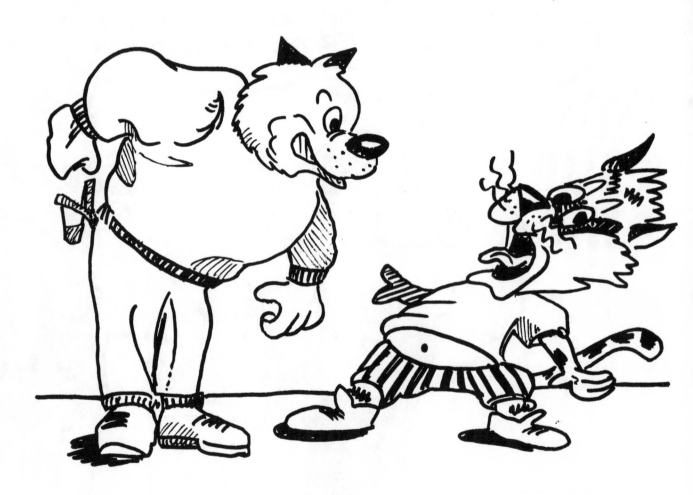

Bear was getting so far behind in his reading they had a special teacher come in to help him. One reason he was having so many problems was he was still reversing letters, not just b's and d's but whole words. Bear would say *was*, when the word was *saw*, or he would write *at*, when the word was *that*. Then in the next sentence he would say the words right, or he would write it down right. Bear told the teacher that he knew what the words were, but he would say it wrong, thinking he was saying it right. He didn't understand why he did it. It just happened. The teacher didn't know why either. She wrote a note to Bear's mom, and told her that Bear was not trying hard enough, and that he was not paying attention (at-ten-tion) in class.

That wasn't true. Bear was one of the best dogs in school. He would always listen, so he could hear what the teacher was saying. The only way Bear could learn was by hearing what the teacher said in class. Bear wanted to do well in school, and to become smarter.

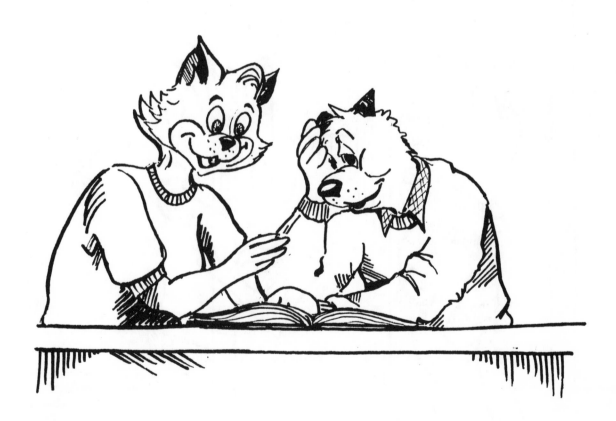

A few years had passed, Bear was now in 8th grade, and he was getting C's and D's in most of his classes. Even though Bear was in the 8th grade, he was only reading at a 2nd grade level, and spelling at a first grade level.

Because Bear was so far behind in his reading, it also affected how well he was doing in his other classes, like English. In English class Bear would write some words down that were misspelled. He would also put words in the sentences that didn't belong. A lot of what Bear was writing didn't make sense, or you couldn't figure out what he was trying to say. Then when Bear tried to read it, to see if he made any mistakes, he couldn't spell or read very well, so he didn't know that he was misspelling words. In English, Bear's grades were D-'s, and F's. That was his hardest class.

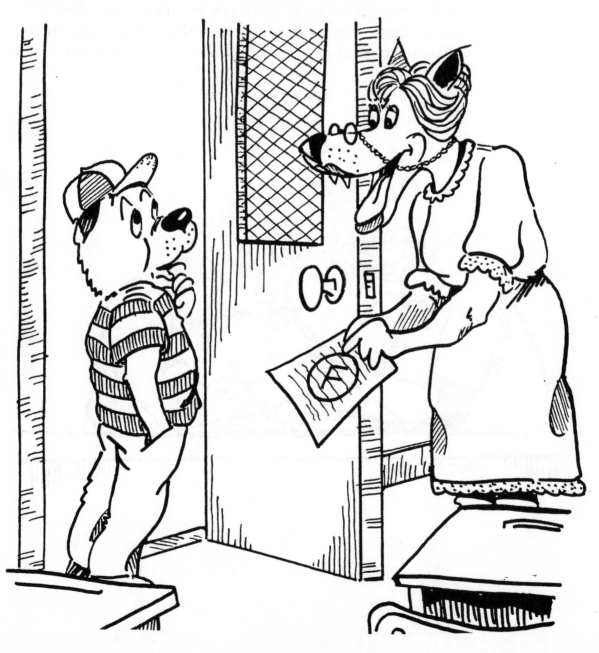

Bear sometimes felt that he was retarded. He felt that was the reason why he couldn't read, spell, or do math very well. That was also why he felt he was doing so poorly in school.

Because Bear wasn't doing very well in school, he felt the other dogs, and cats were making fun of him behide his back. So Bear became very quiet. He hardly had any friends. He felt nobody liked him.

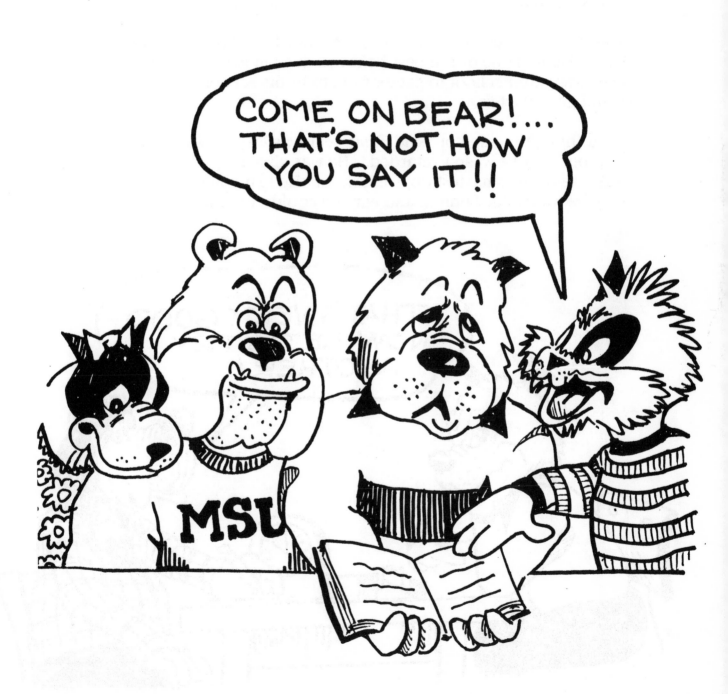

In 8th grade they called Bear to the office to give him an IQ test. They were checking to see if Bear's IQ was lower than the rest of the dogs and cats in his class. If his IQ was lower, they were going to send Bear to a special school to get the extra help he needed.

After the test the doctor was shocked to find out how well Bear did. He told Bear that his IQ was way above normal, and he should be reading and spelling at or above his grade level. The doctor told the school that Bear was lazy, and he was not trying hard enough. He also said that Bear should be one of the smart dogs in school.

That was not true. Bear was trying his hardest; he always was in class. He was one of the best behaved dogs in school. He would even stay after school to get extra help in his school work so he could get smarter.

Even though the doctor "said" that Bear was lazy he was happy to find out that he wasn't retarded. He was also happy to hear that he was one of the smartest dogs in school. He just couldn't understand why he was so far behind, and why he couldn't read.

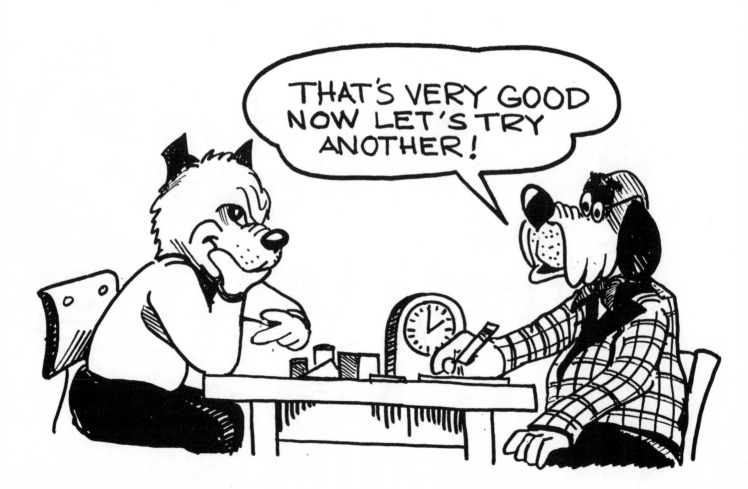

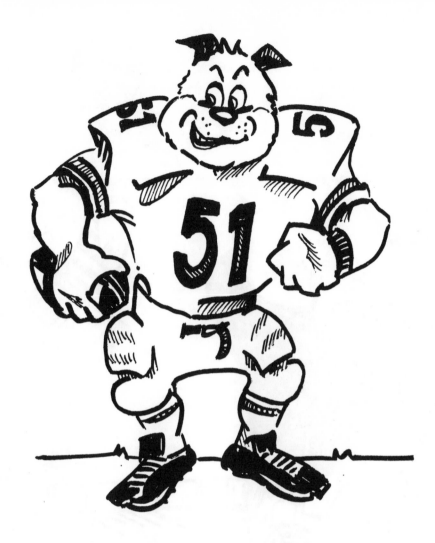

The next year Bear started playing sports in school. He was one of the most talented (tal-ent-ed) athletes (ath-letes) in his class. He became one of the most popular dogs in school. Even though Bear was well liked, he still had a low self-esteem. He wanted to be liked, but he hardly talked to the other dogs because he felt out of place. Some dogs thought he was stuck up. Bear was just afraid that if the other dogs knew him better, they would find out that he couldn't read, spell, or do math very well and would make fun of him, and call him names. So he kept to himself.

Three more years had passed, and Bear made it to the 12th grade still not knowing how to read. His reading level moved up to the 3rd grade level.

Halfway through the year, Bear knew that the teachers were letting him pass. Bear felt that school was a waste of time, so he dropped out only a half a credit short of graduating (grad-u-ate-ing). Bear started working thinking he didn't need a good education.

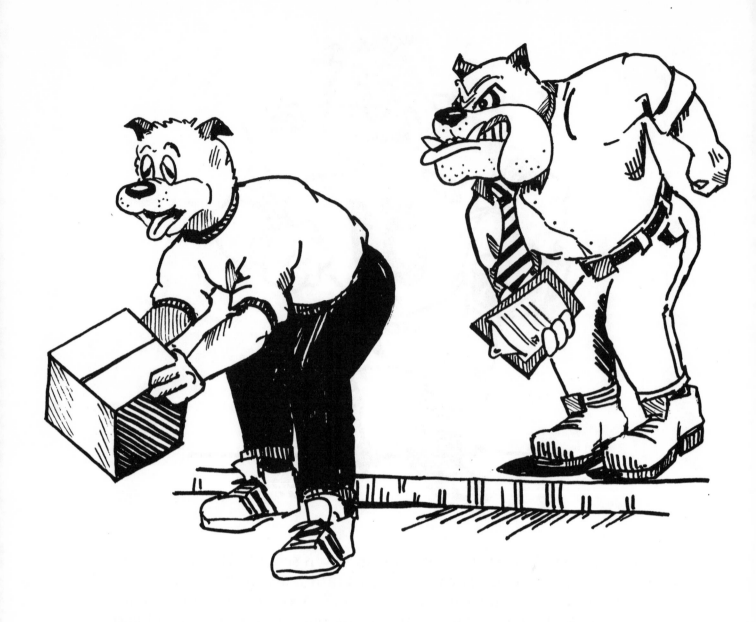

It didn't take long for Bear to see how important (im-por-tant)
school was. The jobs he was getting were jobs for dogs that had
very little ambition (am-bi-tion) in life. The jobs were not
challenging (chal-lenge-ing) enough for him. Bear wanted to show
his boss how intelligent (in-tel-li-gent)he was. His bosses treated
Bear like he had a brain of a two year old. Bear didn't like that.
Bear liked doing things on his own. He liked solving problems. He
wanted to learn.

What Bear learned was how important school really was. It also was
important to have a good education, if you want other dogs and cats
to value your opinion. Bear wanted other dogs and cats to look up
to him. In order for that to happen, he needed a education.

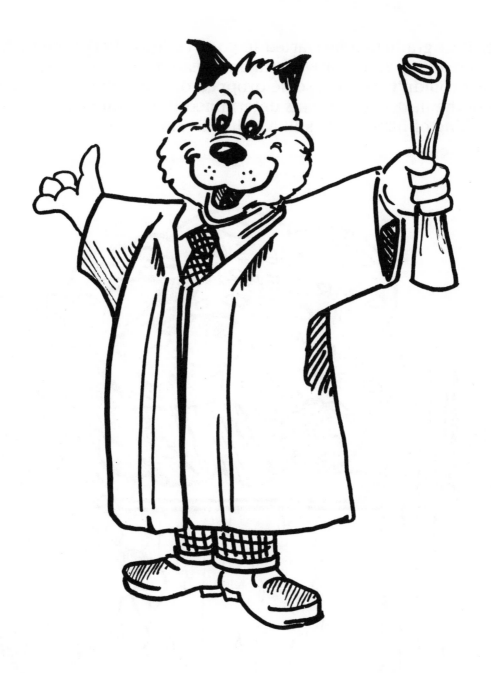

That summer Bear went to summer school and graduated from high school. He wanted other dogs to think that he was smart and if he stayed on those other jobs they would think he had no ambition in life.

After Bear graduated he started to go to college. In college he had lots of reading, and Bear was still only reading at a 3rd grade level. He just couldn't keep up, so he dropped out, and then went back to school the next year. He was determined (de-ter-mined) to make something of himself. He still had his dream, to become famous.

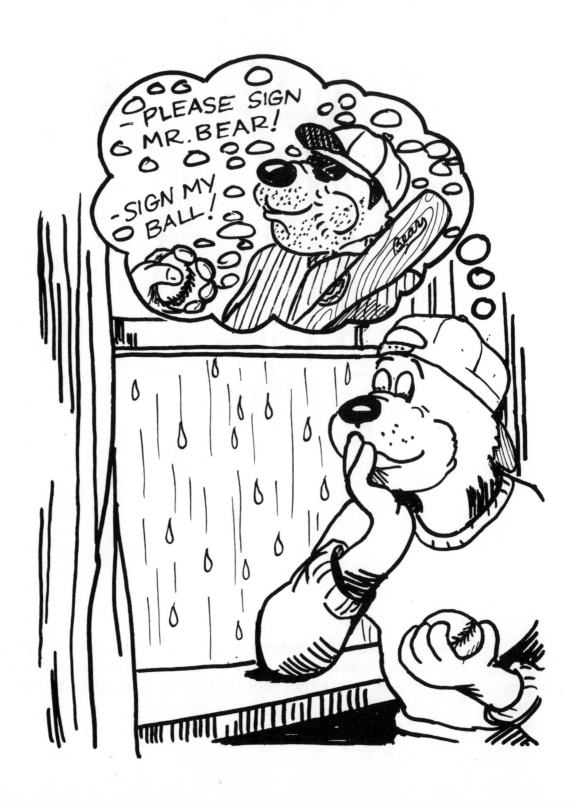

Bear would keep on dropping out and going back to school trying to pass the same classes, English and Math. He did that for two and a half years. He took a total of 18 classes, and only passed 6 of them, and the classes he passed had to do with art and sports. These were the two things at which he was very good. He never passed English or Math.

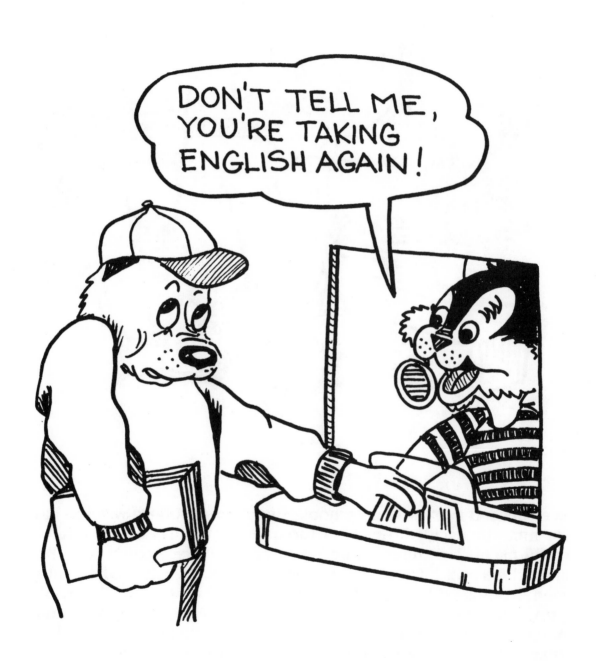

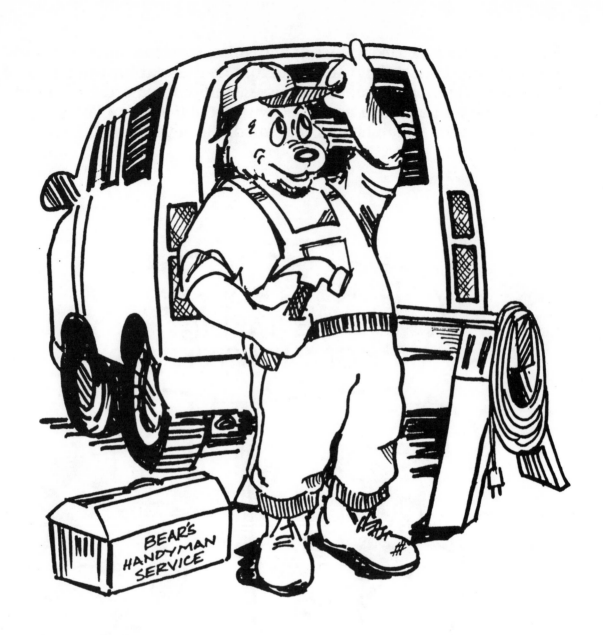

Bear needed a break from school. He saw that college was too hard for him. He decided (de-cid-ed) to quit for a year, and see if he could make something of himself without a college education. Bear started his own business doing home repairs. He was making lots of money doing odd jobs, but he knew he could do better. He wasn't using his mind like he liked and he would not become famous doing home repairs. He went back to school and took English again. He knew this was his worst subject, but he also knew that it was very important if he wanted to graduate from college. This was the sixth time Bear took English in college.

The teacher asked the class to write a paper on whatever they wanted, and to make it two pages long. They had three days to work on it. Bear wanted to do good on this paper. He knew he had to pass English in order to stay in college. He worked on it for hours. He even had someone correct his misspelled words. He thought he had done a good job on the paper. He thought the teacher would give him a B- to a C on the paper. He couldn't wait to get it back.

A few days later they got their papers back. When Bear saw what his grade was he was crushed. He got an F on it, and the teacher wanted to see him after class. He told Bear that was the worst paper he had ever seen, and that he would never become a writer. He said that Bear should drop out of his class, and go back to elementary (el-e-men-ta-ry) school. Bear was almost in tears. He couldn't believe that someone could be so mean and say that.

That was the last time Bear went to college. He knew now that he would have to figure out some other way to get an education.

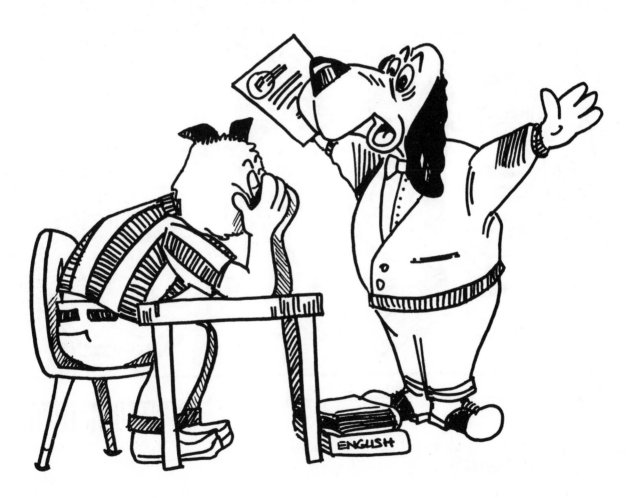

Bear would watch all the educational (ed-u-ca-tion-al)shows he could. He would ask successful (suc-cess-ful)dogs how they got to be such good business dogs. He learned all he could about running a business. He found out that hard work, not giving up, and being honest were the most important things in running a business. The home repair business was doing great. Bear had more work than he knew what to do with. But Bear wanted to do more with his life. He had a deep feeling that he wasn't living up to his full potential (po-ten-tial). He wanted other dogs to admire him for his accomplishments (ac-com-plish-ments) to dog-kind. He wanted to be famous.

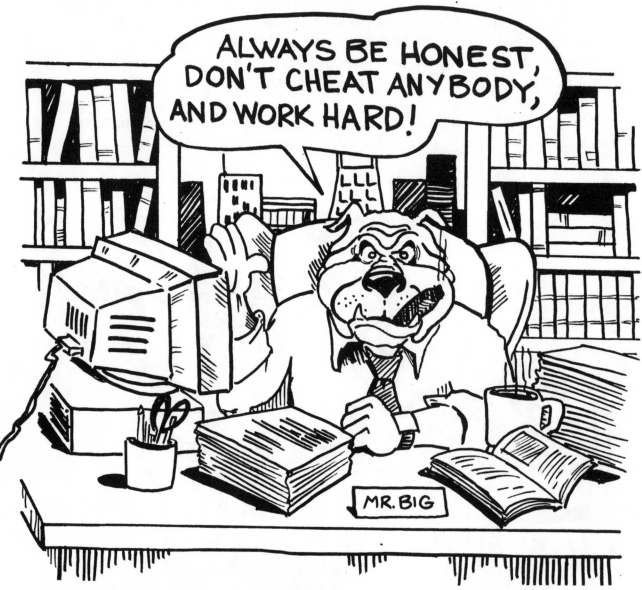

POTENTIAL: capable of becoming actual
ACCOMPLISHMENTS: do, fulfill

He had the chance to buy a business that was more challenging (chal-leng-ing), so he bought a comedy club. He hired a dog that had a slight case of Dyslexia. The dog's name was Kym. Kym started to notice that Bear's handwriting was unreadable, that he couldn't read, and he didn't know how to spell. One day Kym asked Bear if he was Dyslexic. That was the first time Bear heard that word. He didn't know what it was. Kym started telling him all about it-how you reverse letters, and see words that aren't there. How dogs with Dyslexia have messy notes and messy desks and that most dogs with Dyslexia are very smart. She also said that dogs with Dyslexia are good at figuring out different ways of doing things.

It was like she knew all about him. By the time she was done talking, Bear realized that he might have been Dyslexic, and now he understood why he couldn't read, and why he couldn't spell. It wasn't because he was dumb. It was because he had Dyslexia.

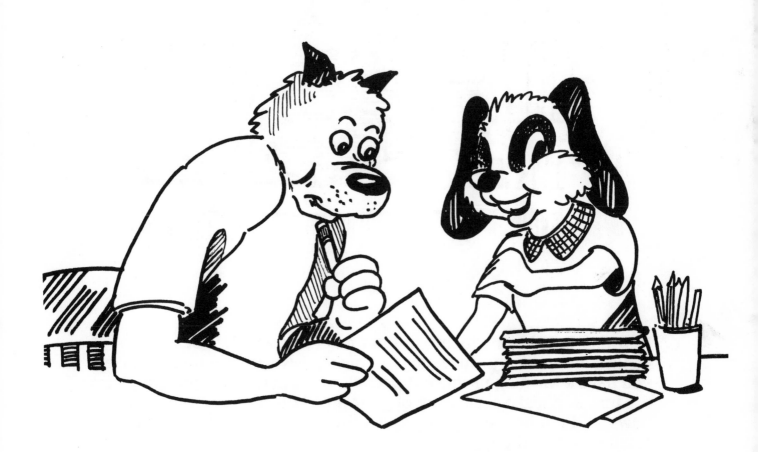

Bear started to talk to other dogs about it, so he could understand what Dyslexia was. The first thing he wanted to know was if you can overcome this learning problem. He found out that you can never overcome Dyslexia. You will always have it. You have to learn how to cope with it, and how to get around it by doing things in a different way. By now Bear was very good at learning different ways of doing things. He did it all his life. You become very creative (cre-ate-tive)in solving problems when you have Dyslexia.

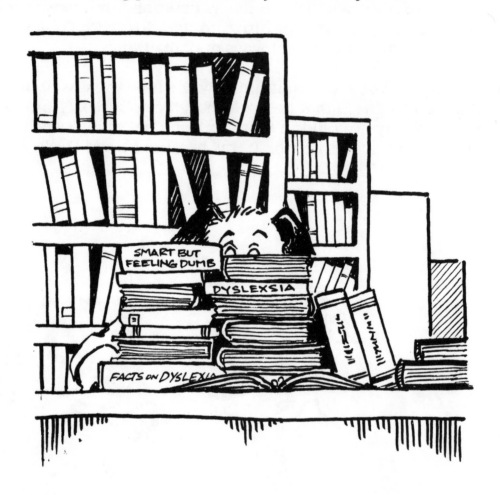

Now that Bear knew why he couldn't read, and why he got F's in English, he wanted to show dogs all over the world that just because you have a learning problem it doesn't mean that you can't live your dreams, and make something of your life. You can overcome your flaws, and not be the dog they call a dummy. He wanted to show smaller dogs and puppies that you can fight it. So Bear went back to the one thing he hated to do. That was writing, Bear wanted to write a book. He knew this was his way to become famous.

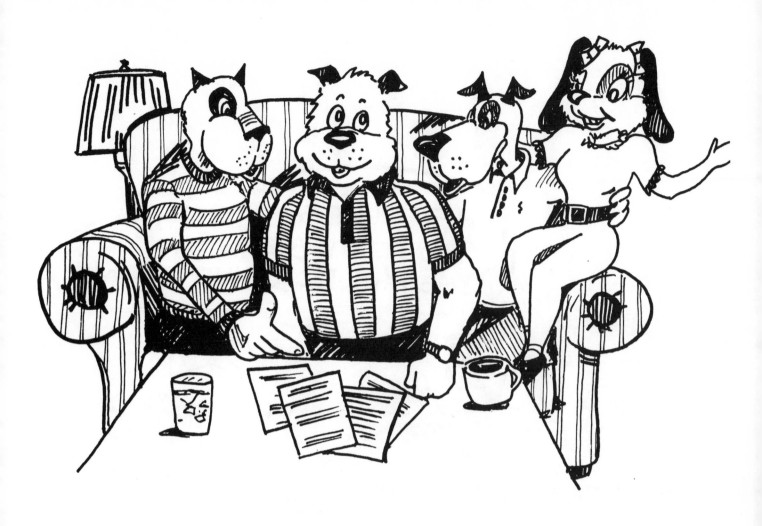

Bear sat down, and started to write. He would write a little each day until he was done. Then he would show it to his dog friends, and they would howl at it. But Bear was not going to let that stop him. He would write it again, and again, and his friends would howl some more, but Bear would not give up. He rewrote it until he got it right. He wrote it over 20 times, and it was done. It was ready to go to the printer. It took Bear over three years to write his first book. He wanted to show the world that just because you are Dyslexic, and you can't do things like normal dogs, it doesn't mean you can't do it. You just have to do it a little differently, and keep on trying. One day you will make it over that wall, and show everyone you can do it, and that you are no different than them, and that you are smart!

The book was printed and sold thousands of copies. Dogs all over the world wanted to hear Bear's story about how he overcame Dyslexia.

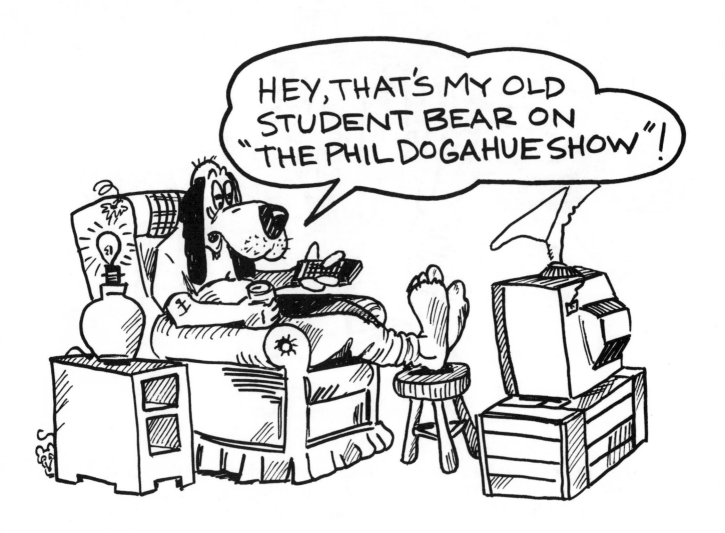

Today, Bear has four books published and he has been written up in 100's of newspapers and magazines around the country. He appeared on the Donahue show and 1000's of other TV and radio shows. He is also planning to go back to college. Bear plans on passing English, and getting his degree in therapy (ther-a-py).

If you are a kid that has Dyslexia you can overcome it just like Bear did. You just have to believe in yourself, and keep trying. One day you can make your dreams come true just like Bear did. You just have to keep on trying and not give up. If Albert Einstein had listened to the kids that made fun of him, he would have never become the great scientist he was. Yes, Albert Einstein was Dyslexic, and when Albert Einstein was in school they put him in a corner with a dunce cap on.

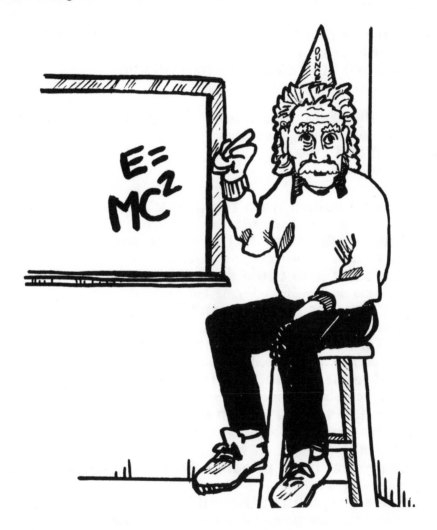

These stories were based on a real person, the author of this book, and all of the things happened to him. Today he still gets letters back that he had written to newspapers that make fun of the way he writes, but he doesn't let that stop him from doing what he likes best, and that is helping people overcome their problems. The dog, Bear, was Barry's dog, and best friend. Barry used Bear's name to keep his dog's name in memory of him. Bear died on Aug. 11, 1994. Bear was 14 years old.

The top and bigger letters has been edited and the bottom in smaller letters is the real way Barry writes.

A little more about the author and his dyslexia:
A little more about the author and his dislexea

Barry Rosen was born in St. Louis, Missouri, on November 22,
Barry Rosen was born in St. Louis Mosirey, on Novmerber 22
1959. He graduated high school in 1978 from Parkway North in
1959. He graduated high shcool in 1978 form parkway north in
St . Louis where he lived for 26 years. He moved to Knoxville,
St. Louis were he lifed for 26 years. He moved to Knoxville
Tennessee on June 5, 1986 where he still lives.
Tennasee on June 5 1986 where he still lives.

Barry also has dyslexia, which was the reason behind this book,
Barry also has dislexia witch is the reason behide his book
"The Dog That Didn't Give Up."
The dog that didn't give up.

The word dyslexia comes from the Greek and means reading
The word dislexia comes from the greeks and meaings reading
difficulty or word blindness. In the 1800s, the word was used
diffacuttea or word blindness in the 1800's the word was used
to describe an adult who could read at one time, but, due to a
to discribe an audat who could read at one time but due to a
head injury or gunshot wound to the head during battle, forgot
head injerrey or gunshot woune to the head during battle for got
how to read. Today, doctors know more about dyslexia. They
how to read. Today doctors know more about dislexia they
now know that most people inherit the disorder from one
now know that most people inherrat the disorder from one
parent or have had some problem during childbirth.
perant or have problems dering childbirth. It is also known that

It is also known that most people who have dyslexia barely have
most people with dislexia bearly have
any noticeable signs, while others like Barry are severe cases.
eneey noitisable signs while ether people like Barry are siever cases.
Of the people who have dyslexia, one in 10 are severe cases, and
Of the people who have dislexia one in ten are server cases and
nine out of 10 are boys. The most common thing you hear about
nine out of ten are boys.

a person with dyslexia is they reverse letters or words, but that
The most commom thing you here about a person with dislexia is thay revers letters or words but that
is only a small part of it.
is only a small part of it.

In Barry's case he reverses letters and words. He also puts
In Barrys case he revers letters and words he also puts

letters that don't belong in words or mispell words. Barry also
letters at don't belong in word or misspell words Barry also

has a hard time blending sounds together. His dyslexia
has a hard time blending sounds together his dislexia

fluctuates and his reading and spelling levels change daily.
fulkuate and his reading and spelling level change daily. Barry also has to witch

Barry also has to watch his diet. In some people, the food they
his diet in some people the food thay

eat makes the disorder worse. It can lower your IQ and drop
eat makes the disorder wrost it can lower your IQ and drop

your grade level as mush as one or two grades., depending on
your grade leavel as much as one or two grade depending on

your sugar intake. One or two grade levels to a person who's
your suger intake. One or two grade leavals to a person who is

reading at a 4th-or 5th-grade level is a lot. (*If you need more*
reading that a 4th or 5th grade level is a lot (If you need more

information on food intake and dyslexia, is
information on food intakeand information on dislexia is

included at the end of the book.)
includedthat the end of the book.)

Barry was 26 when he found out he was dyslexic, and didn't
Barry was 26 when he fornd out he was dislexia and didn't

learn about food intake until he was 32. He now knows how he is
learn about food intake intill he was 32 he now knows how he is

affected by eating the wrong foods. Words move around on the
afated by eating the wrong foods.Words move around on the

page, he has a hard time focusing on letters and he forgets what
page he has a hard time focusing on letters and he forget what

some letters look like. It's not unusual for him to forget what he
some letters look like it not unsueall of him to forget what he

just read, either.
just read eather

While doing research for this book, Barry also learned that one in
While doing recheach on the book Barry also leand that one in

seven people have some form of dyslexia, and that there are
seven people have some form of dislexia and that there are

over 100 different types of the disorder, according to Dr. Peter
over 100 different tipes of the disorder accornding to Dr. Peter

Winograd of the University of Kentucky, and no two people
Winograd of the Univeratey of Katucky and know two people

have the same symptoms.
have the same simtims.

Today, Barry is living his dream, touring the country promoting
Today Barry is liveing his dream touring the country promoting

his books: "250 Ways To Be Romantic," "Marriage 101:Back to the
his book 250 Ways To Be Romanctic Marriage 101 Back to the
Basics," and "The Dog That Didn't Give Up." In addition to
basics and I'm not stubut I'm dislexif in addischin to
traveling the country speaking to kids and adults, he also owns a
travling the country speaking to kids and adults he also owns a
publishing company and teaches people how to get on radio and
publishing company and teaches people how to get on radio and
television and to get write-ups in magazines and newspapers.
Telavition and gets write ups in magazines and newspapers

Barry has appeared on over 1000 radio and television shows like
Barry has appeared on over 1000 radio and telavion shows like
The Donahue show, Charles Perez show and has been
The donahue show and charle preaz show and has been
interviewed in hundreds of magazines and newspapers around
interviewed in hunreds of magazines and newspapers around
the country.

When Barry is not on the road with his two dogs, Bear Jr.-- the
the country. When Barry is not on the road with his two dogs Bear Jr.
the son of Bear and Romeo, he buys old houses and restores
the son of Bear and Rommeo. He buys old houses and restore
them for fun. Other Hobbies include fishing, hiking, caving,
them for fun.

collecting rocks and old cameras, camping, scuba diving and
Other hoppies include fishing hiking caving colecting rocks and old camras camping scaba diving ang
going to auctions.
going to alctions.

Barry is happy that he is dyslexic, and that he has gone through
Barry is happy that he is dislexia and that he has gone thought
all the hard times, because it made him who he is today. If he
all the hard times because it made him who he is today. If he
had to do it all over again, he would only change one thing: he
had to do it all over again he would only change one thing. He
would have not skiped the last half of his senior year of high
would of not skip the last half of his serorir year in high
school.
school.

Barry hopes these books will help you to see that if you believe
Barry hopes these book will help you to beleave
in your dreams, you can do what ever you want, all you have to
you can do what every you went all you have to do is beleave in
do is believe in yourself and your dreams will come true. If your
your dream and if your dream doen't come true it wasn't a

dream doesn't come true it wasn't a dream it was a wish. You
dream it was a wish. Keep tring and don't give up.
should never give up on a dream.

**To contact Barry or to schedule an interview, or lecture, call
(432) 691-1990 or write: B.R. Publishing Co., 1725 Pinebrook Dr.,
Knoxville, TN. 37909**

A little more about the author and about his Dyslexia.

Barry was born in St. Louis Missouri on November, 22 1959. He
graduated high school in 1978 from Parkway North in St. Louis, were [*where*]
he lived for 26 years. He move to Knoxville, Tennessee on June, 5 [*moved*] [*Tenn.*]
1986, where he still lives.

While doing research on the book, Barry learn that one in seven and [*ed*] [*to*]
half people have some form of Dyslexia, and that there are over 100
different types of Dyslexia, according to Dr. Peter Winograd of the
University of Kentucky. There are severe different forms of Dyslexia, [*several*]
raging from seeing words backwards to seeing words jumping off
the paper. Most people that have Dyslexia barely have any [*who*]
noticeable signs, and other like Barry are severe. The people that [*while*] [*who*] [*lowercase*]
have Dyslexia, 1 in 10 are server and 9 out of 10 are boys. The most [*cases*]
common thing you hear about a person with Dyslexia is that they
reveres letter or words, but that is only a small part of it.

The word Dyslexia comes from the Greeks, meaning reading
difficulty or word blindness.

In the 1800's the word was use to decribe an adults that could read [*1800s*] [*used*] [*who*]
at one time, but us to a head injury or a gunshot wound to the head [*due*]
from battle, forgot how to read. Today, doctors know more about [*during*]
it. They now know that most people inherited from one parent or
have some problems with their child birth. [*had*] [*during*] [*the disorder*]

Leads talk about Barry and what kind of Dyslexia he has. Remember
that you or your kids may have a different from of Dyslexia. In [*form*]
Barry's case he reveres letter and words. He also puts letter in words [*reverses*]
that doesn't belong or he will put a words in sentence misspelling it [*don't*] [*misspelling*]
but spelling a word right that is the wrong word. Then when you
read it, it doesn't make sense. Barry also has a hard time blending
the sounds together. The last thing is Barry, Dyslexia will fluctuate. [*Finally*]
But is reading and spelling level will change daily it depends on what [*His*]
he has eaten that day. In some people the food you eat can make it
worse like it does for Barry. It can lower your IQ and drop your

[handwritten margin notes: New Paragraph; (2 graphs) his graph sould be moved higher; who is Leads?]

New graph ↑

reading level as much as one or to grade levels depending on ~~how~~ *the amount of* ~~much lactose you eat or drink.~~ *consumed* One or two grade ~~levels~~ to a person who is reading at a 4th or 5th grade level is a lot. (If you need more information on food, there will be a list of information you can order to help you learn more about Dyslexia at the end of this book.)

Barry was 26 when he found out he was ~~Dyslexia~~ *dyslexic,* and he didn't learn about how food can make it worse till he was 32. ~~What happen to~~ *When* Barry ~~when he~~ eats the wrong foods ~~then he tries to read or write is. The~~ words will move around on the paper. He has a hard time focusing on letters and ~~he will~~ forget what some letters look like or he will forget what he just read.

But I Today, Barry is living his dream, touring the country promoting his books "250 Ways to be Romantic," "Marriage 101" "Back To the Basics," and "I'm not stupid I'm Dyslexic!" Going to schools all over the country doing talks for kids and adults ~~just like you.~~ He also ~~ownes~~ *owns* his own publishing ~~co.~~ *company* and ~~teachs~~ *teaches* people how to get on Radio & ~~TV~~ *television* and get write ups in magazines and Newspapers. Barry has ~~appearing~~ *appeared* on over 1000 radio an TV shows like ~~the~~ Donhue, and has been ~~written up~~ *interviewed* in ~~100's~~ *hundreds* of magazines and newspapers around the country.

When Barry is not on the road with his two dogs Bear Jr., the son of Bear and Romemeo, He buys old houses and restores them for fun, some other ~~hobbies of Barry's~~ are Fishing, Hicking, caving, ~~colleting~~ *collecting* rocks, camping, ~~colleting old camras,~~ *and old cameras* ~~squba~~ *scuba* diving, and going to ~~ations~~ *auctions.*

Barry is so happy that he is ~~Dyslexia~~ *dyslexic* and that he went ~~thought~~ *through* all the hard times, Because it made ~~them~~ *him* who he is today. If he had to do it all over again he would only change one thing ~~and that is he~~ ~~graduat~~ *finished his senior year of high school* ~~wouldn't of drop out of school in 12th grade.~~

These are some of Barry press release he sent out and got back. Barry still has people make fun of his writing and he still will not give up his dream and that is to learn all he can and not to give up.

Barry hopes these book help you see that if you ~~beleave~~ *believe* you can do *anything* it and you see your self doing it, you can do what ever you ~~went~~ *want.* you just have to ~~beleave~~ *believe* in yourself.

If you would like to write or contact Barry and tell him you story or how this book help you, or if you would like to book Barry for ~~a talk~~ *an interview* ~~you can~~ call him at (615)691-1990 or write him at B. R, Publishing Co. 1725 Pinebrook Dr. Knoxville, TN 37909

TEACHER GUIDE

1) Why were the other dogs and cats howling at Bear?
_____
_____

2) Which paw did Bear use when saying the Pledge of Allegiance? Right____ Left____

3)Why would Bear get in fights? _____
_____
_____

4)In English , Bear grades were? A's__ B's__ C's__ D's__ F's__

5)When Bear had a IQ test, what did the doctor say was wrong with Bear?
_____
_____
_____

6)What grade level was Bear reading at in the 12th grade?
_____

7)How many times did Bear take English in college?
_____

8) How old was Bear when He found out he was Dyslexia?
_____

9)How many times did Bear rewrite the book? _____

10) What famous scientist had Dyslexia? _____
_____

SPECIAL THANKS TO THESE PEOPLE FOR HELPING ME

Kym Lain for helping me from day one reading my first copy
Dorian Lain helping me read my first copy
Brian Lain reading the book and telling me what to change
Margaret Parker for having a child reading the book and proof-reading the final copy
Bearden Hill Elementary School for reading the book and telling me what to change and their teacher
Ms. Darlene Neuhaus The kid's names are Caroline Broome, Lee Robinson, Adrienne Rogers, William
Young, Jessica Heldman, Brian L. Griffith, Anna West-Hammer, Scott Lawson, Carrie Hemsley, Preston
Ralston, Rachel Royer, Sarah Rogers, Rebecca Drumm, Kate Gutekunst, Rachel Casey, Will Haslam,
Deena Goldstein, Megas Locke, Ross Cox, Kasra Taleb-Haghipoor, Michael Currier, Packer Wright III
West Hill Elementary School for reading the book and telling me they like the book the way it was..

NEWSLETTER AND MORE INFORMATION ON DYSLEXIA

NEWSLETTER COST AND S&H

1)THE DEFINITION OF DYSLEXIA	$1.00 plus .35
2)THE HISTORY OF DYSLEXIA	$1.00 plus .35
3)WHAT CAUSES DYSLEXIA & HOW DO YOU GET IT	$2.00 plus .65
4)WHAT ARE THE THEORIES ON CURING DYSLEXIA	$2.00 plus .65
5)WHAT ARE THE SIGNS OF DYSLEXIA	$2.00 plus .65
6)FAMOUS PEOPLE WHO HAVE DYSLEXIA	$1.00 plus .35
7)FOODS THAT ARE GOOD AND BAD FOR YOU	$2.75 plus .95
8)THE DRUGS AND THEIR SIDE EFFECTS	$1.25 plus .35
9)THE LAWS (very important)	$2.00 plus .65
10)WHAT ARE THE TESTS YOU TAKE FOR DYSLEXIA	$2.00 plus .65
11)SCHOOLS & ORGANIZATIONS FOR DYSLEXIA	$3.00 plus .95
12)BOOKS ON DYSLEXIA	$1.50 plus .65
13)NEWSPAPER ARTICLES	$1.50 plus .85
ALL NEWSLETTERS	$15.00 plus $3.00

MOTIVATION TALK FOR KIDS IS AVAILABLE ON
AUDIO CASSETTE TAPE $7.95 plus .95

SEND CHECK OR MONEY ORDER TO 1725 PINEBROOK DR. KNOXVILLE TN 37909